Easy 6-minutes Exercise for Fitness at 60+

Simple home exercises to boost your strength and health.

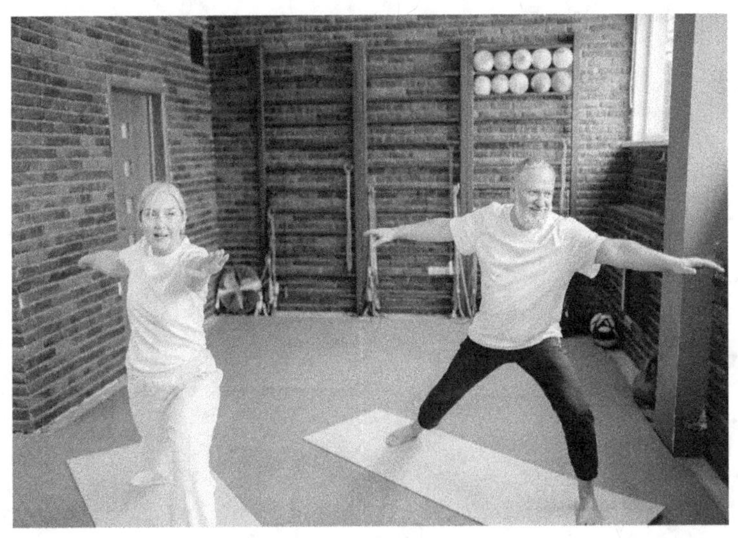

Clark Leonard

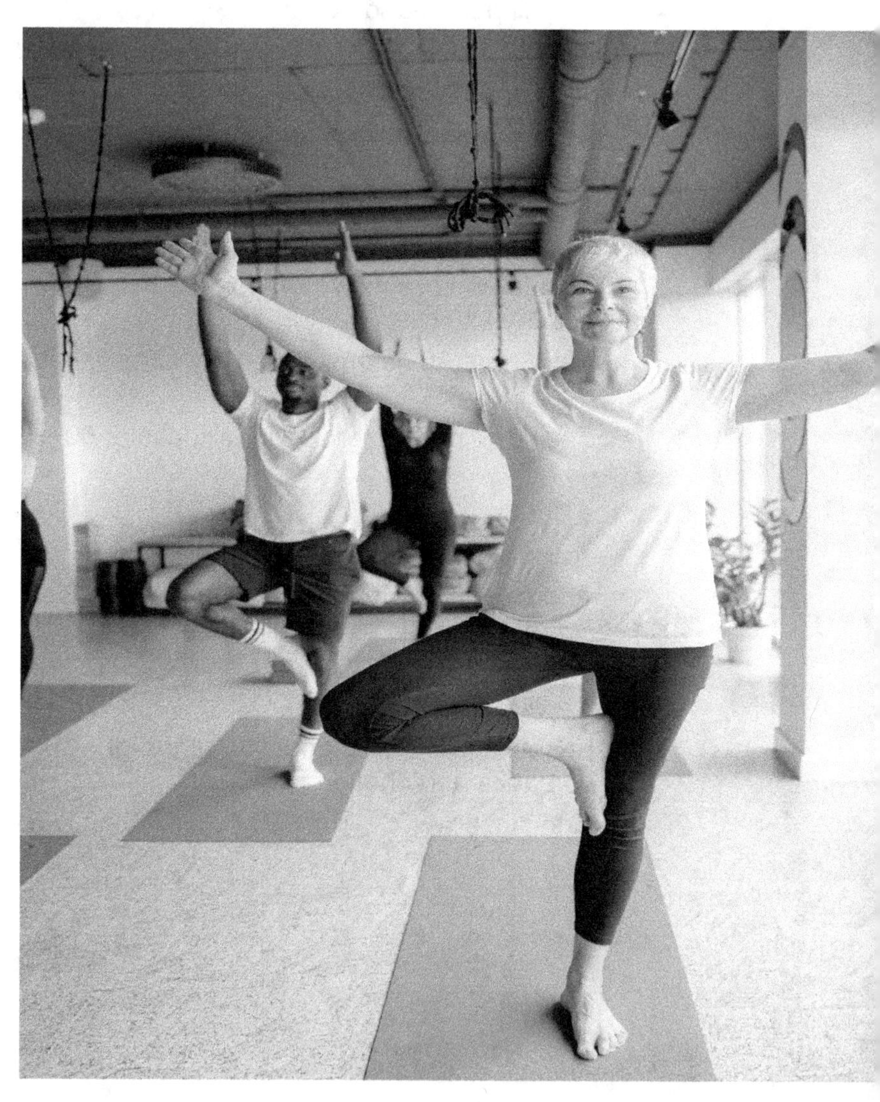

INTRODUCTION

The aging process often brings about changes in the body, such as decreased muscle mass, joint stiffness, and reduced flexibility. However, the benefits of physical activity on mental, cardiovascular, and musculoskeletal health are well-established. Recognizing the unique needs of individuals in their 60s and beyond, the Easy 6-Minute Exercise for fitness at 60+ aims to provide a manageable and enjoyable way for seniors to incorporate fitness into their daily lives.

This exercise routine is specifically tailored to address the concerns of older adults, emphasizing safety, simplicity, and adaptability. It acknowledges the diverse range of abilities and health conditions within senior demographic, making it accessible to those with varying fitness levels and mobility challenges. The ultimate goal is to boost strength, good health, promote longevity, independence, and a higher quality of life through regular, manageable physical activity.

As we delve into the details of the Easy 6-Minute Exercise for fitness at 60+ it's important to highlight the evidence supporting the positive impact of short bursts of exercise on overall health. Research suggests that even brief, moderate-intensity activities can contribute significantly to cardiovascular health, bone density, and mental well-being. This reinforces the idea that exercise doesn't have to be time-consuming to be effective, particularly for seniors seeking to maintain or improve their fitness levels.

In the sections that follow, we will explore the key components of the Easy 6-Minute Exercise for fitness at 60+, including a variety of exercises that target boosting strength, flexibility, and balance. Additionally, we will provide guidelines for proper warm-up and cool-down activities, essential for preventing injuries and ensuring a positive exercise experience. Whether you are new to fitness or looking to revitalize your current routine, this easy-to-follow regimen promises to be a valuable resource on your journey to health and vitality in your 60s and beyond.

Chapter One

Understanding Fitness at 60+

Recognizing the importance of staying active in the senior years.

Staying active in the senior years is crucial for maintaining overall well-being. Regular physical activity has been linked to various health benefits, including improved cardiovascular health, enhanced mobility, and reduced risk of chronic conditions. Engaging in activities like walking, swimming, or gentle exercises helps maintain muscle strength and flexibility. Moreover, staying active promotes mental health by reducing the risk of cognitive decline and boosting mood. Recognizing the importance of an active lifestyle in the senior years is essential for a healthier and more fulfilling aging process.

Addressing common concerns and misconceptions about exercise for older adults.

Addressing common concerns and misconceptions about exercise for older adults is crucial for promoting a healthy and active lifestyle in this demographic. Many older individuals may harbor fears or misunderstandings about engaging in physical activity, leading to potential barriers to adopting an exercise routine. Here, we'll explore some prevalent concerns and misconceptions and provide insights to dispel them.

1.**Misconception:** Aging means avoiding exercise.

Reality: Regular exercise is beneficial for older adults, promoting overall health, mobility, and independence. It helps manage chronic conditions and enhances mental well-being.

2. Concern: Increased risk of injury.

Reality: While there's a potential for injury, proper guidance, and choosing appropriate activities can significantly reduce this risk. Consultation with healthcare professionals and certified trainers is recommended.

3.Misconception: Only vigorous exercise counts.

Reality: Any form of physical activity contributes to health. Low-impact exercises like walking, swimming, or yoga offer substantial benefits and are gentler on aging joints.

4. Concern: Health conditions limit exercise options.

Reality: Many health conditions can be managed or improved with tailored exercise. A personalized approach, considering individual health status, is essential. Always consult a healthcare provider before starting a new exercise program.

5. Misconception: It's too late to start exercising.

Reality: It's never too late to reap the benefits of exercise. Even starting a moderate routine later in life can lead to improved strength, balance, and overall well-being.

6. Concern: Exercise exacerbates arthritis.

Reality: Properly designed exercise programs can alleviate arthritis symptoms by strengthening muscles around joints. Activities like water aerobics or cycling are joint-friendly.

7. Misconception: Slowing down is normal with age.

Reality: While aging involves changes, maintaining physical activity can slow the decline in muscle mass, bone density, and flexibility, helping older adults stay agile and active.

8. Concern: Lack of social engagement in exercise.

Reality: Group classes, community fitness programs, or exercising with friends can provide social interaction, making the experience enjoyable and motivating for older adults.

9. Misconception: Exercise doesn't impact mental health.

Reality: Physical activity has proven benefits for mental health, reducing stress, anxiety, and depression. It also enhances cognitive function, crucial for maintaining mental sharpness in older age.

10. Concern: Exercise is time-consuming.

Reality: Incorporating physical activity into daily routines, even in shorter durations, can yield positive effects. Consistency is key, and small changes can make a significant impact over time.

Exploring the unique benefits of regular physical activity for individuals aged 60 and above.

Exploring the unique benefits of a 6-minute easy exercise routine for individuals aged 60 and above reveals a tailored approach that caters to the specific needs and considerations of this demographic. While the duration is short, the impact on fitness and overall well-being is noteworthy:

1. Time Efficiency: The 6-minute exercise routine is designed to be quick and efficient, making it accessible for individuals with busy schedules or those who may have physical limitations.

2. Cardiovascular Health: Despite its short duration, the routine incorporates cardiovascular exercises, such as brisk walking or low-impact aerobics, contributing to improved heart health and circulation.

3. Joint-Friendly Movements: The exercises are carefully chosen to be gentle on joints, reducing the risk of strain or injury. This is especially beneficial for seniors who may have arthritis or joint-related concerns.

4. Flexibility and Mobility: The routine includes stretching and mobility exercises, enhancing flexibility and promoting joint range of motion. This is crucial for maintaining an active and independent lifestyle.

5. Strength Building: Incorporating simple resistance exercises, such as bodyweight squats or seated leg lifts, the routine aids in maintaining muscle mass and strength, essential for daily activities.

6. Balance and Stability: Specific exercises targeting balance are included to reduce the risk of falls, a significant concern for older individuals. Improved balance contributes to enhanced stability in daily movements.

7. Adaptability: The 6-minute routine can be easily adapted to individual fitness levels and modified based on any existing health conditions. This adaptability ensures inclusivity for a wide range of participants.

8. Mental Well-being: Engaging in regular, brief exercise has positive effects on mental health, contributing to improved mood, reduced stress, and enhanced cognitive function, factors especially relevant for seniors.

9. Social Engagement: Participating in group sessions or classes centered around the 6-minute routine

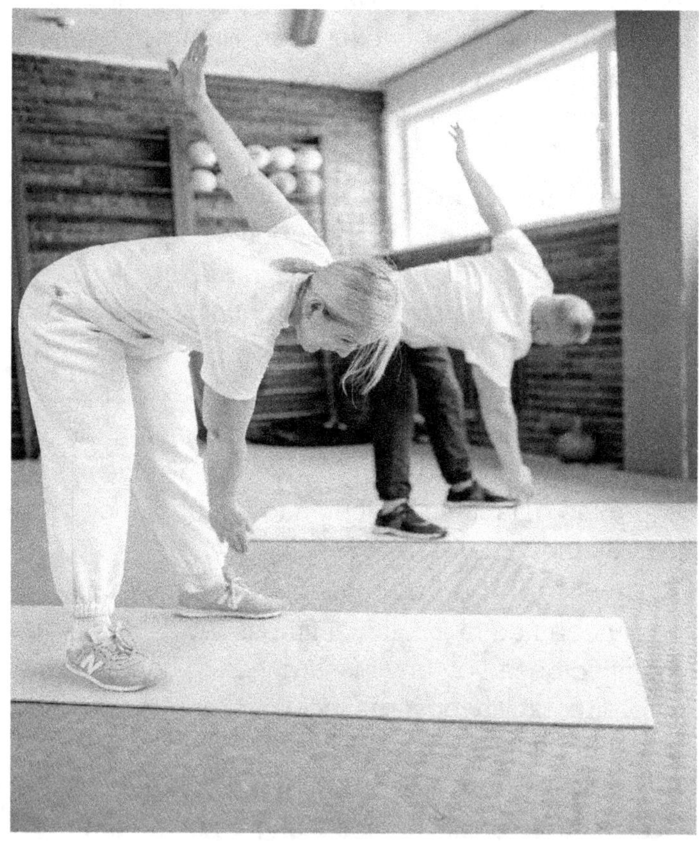

Chapter 2

The Science of 6-Minute Workouts

Delving into the research behind short, efficient exercise routines.

In a fast-paced world where time is a precious commodity, the allure of short, efficient exercise routines has captivated fitness enthusiasts. At the forefront of this movement is the intriguing science behind the 6-minute workout. This comprehensive exploration delves into the research underpinning these brief yet impactful exercise sessions, unraveling the physiological and psychological intricacies that make the 6-minute workout a subject of scientific fascination.

Physiological Responses to Short Exercise Bursts:

Research has illuminated the intricate physiological responses triggered by short bursts of intense exercise, forming the backbone of the 6-minute workout phenomenon. High-intensity interval training

(HIIT), a key component of many 6-minute routines, has been shown to elicit robust metabolic adaptations. The alternation between intense efforts and brief recovery periods challenges the body's energy systems, leading to enhanced cardiovascular function, improved insulin sensitivity, and efficient calorie utilization.

Cellular Adaptations and Molecular Pathways:

At the cellular level, the molecular pathways activated during short, intense exercise sessions provide a deeper understanding of their impact. Studies suggest that brief workouts stimulate the expression of genes associated with mitochondrial biogenesis and oxidative capacity. This not only enhances endurance but also contributes to the overall metabolic health of individuals engaging in 6-minute workouts.

Time-Efficiency and Adherence Factors:

Beyond the physiological realm, the science of 6-minute workouts also considers the practical aspects of incorporating exercise into busy lifestyles. The time-efficiency of these routines aligns with the demands of modern society, offering a viable solution for those seeking effective yet manageable fitness practices. Understanding adherence factors is crucial, as short workouts are more likely to be sustained over the long term, promoting consistent engagement with physical activity.

Psychological Benefits and Mental Well-Being:

The psychological aspects of short, efficient exercise routines play a pivotal role in their popularity. Research indicates that even brief periods of physical activity can positively impact mood, reduce stress, and enhance cognitive function. The accessibility and simplicity of 6-minute workouts contribute to their potential as stress-relievers and mood boosters, making them valuable tools for mental well-being.

Understanding how brief bursts of activity can positively impact cardiovascular health, flexibility, and muscle strength.

The Easy 6-minute Exercise for Fitness at 60+ emphasizes the importance of incorporating short bursts of physical activity into daily routines to promote cardiovascular health, flexibility, and muscle strength in older adults. These brief bursts of activity, even as short as six minutes, can have profound effects on overall fitness.

Cardiovascular health is vital for older adults as it reduces the risk of heart disease, stroke, and other cardiovascular issues. Brief bursts of activity, such as brisk walking, jumping jacks, or stair climbing, help increase heart rate and improve blood circulation. This, in turn, strengthens the heart muscle and enhances its efficiency in pumping blood throughout the body, leading to better cardiovascular health.

Flexibility is another key aspect of fitness, especially for seniors who may experience stiffness and reduced range of motion. Short bursts of activity that involve stretching exercises, yoga poses, or tai chi movements can help improve flexibility by loosening tight muscles and increasing joint mobility. Enhanced flexibility not only aids in daily activities but also reduces the risk of injury from falls and improves overall quality of life.

Muscle strength is crucial for maintaining functional independence and preventing age-related muscle loss (sarcopenia). Brief bouts of strength-training exercises, such as bodyweight squats, push-ups, or resistance band exercises, stimulate muscle growth and development. These activities help older adults maintain muscle mass, improve balance, and support bone health, reducing the risk of fractures and osteoporosis.

Incorporating easy-to-follow, short-duration exercises tailored for seniors can make fitness more accessible and manageable, encouraging consistent participation. By integrating these brief bursts of activity into their daily routines, older adults can experience significant improvements in cardiovascular health, flexibility, and muscle strength, ultimately leading to a healthier and more active lifestyle.

Exploring the concept of interval training for older adults.

Interval training for older adults, as highlighted in the "Easy 6-Minute Exercise for Fitness at 60+" program, offers a tailored approach to fitness that acknowledges the unique needs and capabilities of this demographic. Unlike traditional continuous exercise, interval training allows older adults to achieve similar or even greater fitness gains in a shorter amount of time.

The concept behind interval training involves alternating between periods of higher intensity exercise and periods of lower intensity or rest. For example, a session might consist of alternating between brisk walking and gentle stretching exercises. This approach not only provides variety to the workout but also allows for brief recovery periods, reducing the risk of overexertion and injury.

Research suggests that interval training can be particularly effective for older adults in improving cardiovascular health, increasing muscle strength, and enhancing overall fitness levels. Additionally, interval training has been shown to boost metabolism and improve insulin sensitivity, which can be beneficial for managing weight and reducing the risk of chronic diseases such as type 2 diabetes.

Moreover, interval training can be easily adapted to accommodate individual fitness levels and preferences. Older adults can adjust the intensity and duration of the intervals based on their current fitness level, gradually increasing the challenge as they progress. This flexibility makes interval training accessible to a wide range of older adults, regardless of their starting point.

Overall, exploring the concept of interval training for older adults, as presented in the "Easy 6-Minute Exercise for Fitness at 60+" program, offers a promising approach to promoting health and well-being in this demographic. By incorporating intervals into their exercise routine, older adults can enjoy the benefits of improved fitness and vitality in a safe, efficient, and enjoyable manner.

Chapter Three

Setting the foundation

Preparing the body for exercise with gentle warm-up routines.

Gentle Warm-Up Routines for Preparing the Body for Exercise: A Guide for Fitness at 60+

As individuals age, the importance of a proper warm-up routine before exercise becomes increasingly crucial for maintaining flexibility, preventing injury, and optimizing performance. For those aged 60 and above, incorporating gentle warm-up exercises tailored to their needs is essential. In line with the principles of the Easy 6-Minute Exercise for Fitness at 60+, this guide provides precise instructions on preparing the body effectively for physical activity.

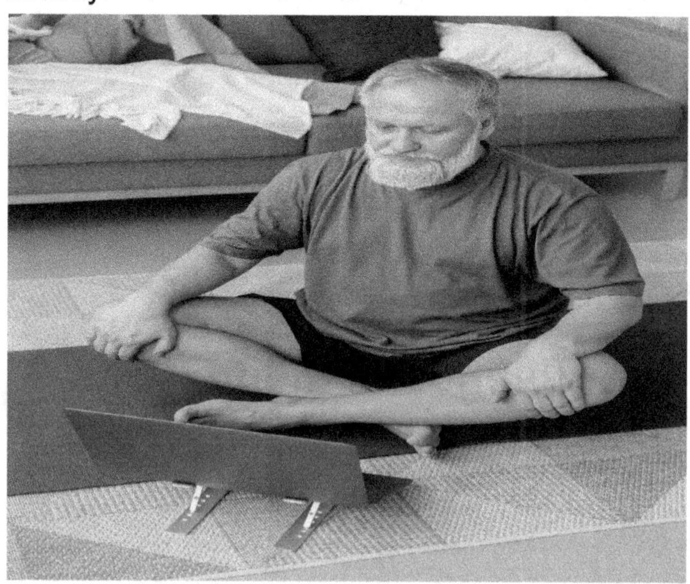

1. **Understanding the Importance of Warm-Up:** With advancing age, the body's flexibility, muscle elasticity, and joint mobility tend to decrease, making it more susceptible to strains, sprains, and other injuries during exercise. A well-designed warm-up routine helps increase blood flow to muscles, elevates body temperature, enhances joint lubrication, and primes the cardiovascular system for physical exertion.

2. **Components of a Gentle Warm-Up Routine:**

a. Joint Mobilization: Begin by gently moving each joint through its full range of motion to lubricate the joints and improve flexibility. Focus on movements such as shoulder circles, neck rotations, arm swings, hip circles, knee lifts, and ankle rolls.

b. Dynamic Stretching: Perform dynamic stretches that target major muscle groups, focusing on movements that mimic those in the upcoming exercise session. Examples include leg swings, arm circles, torso twists, and side bends.

c. Cardiovascular Activation: Incorporate low-intensity cardiovascular exercises to gradually increase heart rate and blood flow.

Options include marching in place, gentle jogging on the spot, or brisk walking.

3. Easy 6-Minute Exercise Warm-Up Routine:

Duration: Aim for approximately 6 minutes to adequately prepare the body for activity without causing fatigue.

Sequence:

1. Begin with 1-2 minutes of joint mobilization exercises, spending 15-30 seconds on each joint.
2. Follow with 2-3 minutes of dynamic stretching, performing 8-10 repetitions of each movement.
3. Conclude with 1-2 minutes of low-impact cardiovascular exercises, gradually increasing intensity.

4. Tips for Safe and Effective Warm-Up:
- Start gradually and progress slowly, listening to your body and avoiding any movements that cause discomfort or pain.
- Maintain proper posture and alignment throughout the warm-up routine, focusing on smooth, controlled movements.

- Incorporate deep breathing exercises to oxygenate the muscles and promote relaxation.

- Stay hydrated before, during, and after the warm-up to support optimal performance and recovery.

Tips on creating a suitable and safe exercise space at home

Creating a suitable and safe exercise space at home for easy 6-minute exercises for fitness at 60+:

1. Clear the area: Remove clutter and obstacles to create a spacious environment free from tripping hazards.
2. Choose appropriate flooring: Opt for non-slip surfaces to prevent falls, such as rubber mats or carpeting.
3. Proper lighting: Ensure adequate lighting to see clearly and avoid accidents during workouts.
4. Sturdy furniture: Use stable chairs or countertops for support during exercises like squats or balance work.

5. Accessibility: Arrange equipment and props within easy reach to minimize strain and promote independence.

6. Safety equipment: Keep a first aid kit nearby and have emergency contacts readily available for peace of mind.

Understanding individual fitness levels and setting realistic goals.

Understanding individual fitness levels is essential for tailoring exercise programs to suit the needs and capabilities of those aged 60 and above. It involves assessing factors such as mobility, strength, flexibility, and cardiovascular health. By understanding where one stands in terms of fitness, individuals can set realistic goals that align with their current abilities and health conditions.

When it comes to setting goals inline with the Easy 6-Minute Exercise for Fitness at 60+, it's important to start small and gradually increase intensity and duration as progress is made. Realistic goals may include improving balance, increasing flexibility, building strength, or enhancing cardiovascular endurance. These objectives must be time-bound, meaningful, quantifiable, achievable, and targeted (SMART).

For example, a realistic goal could be to perform the Easy 6-Minute Exercise routine three times a week for four weeks, gradually increasing the number of repetitions or duration of each exercise as tolerated. Additionally, goals should be personalized to accommodate individual preferences, limitations, and health considerations.

By setting realistic goals and gradually progressing towards them, individuals can improve their overall fitness, enhance their quality of life, and reduce the risk of age-related health issues. Consistency, patience, and listening to one's body are key principles to keep in mind when pursuing fitness goals at any age, especially for older adults.

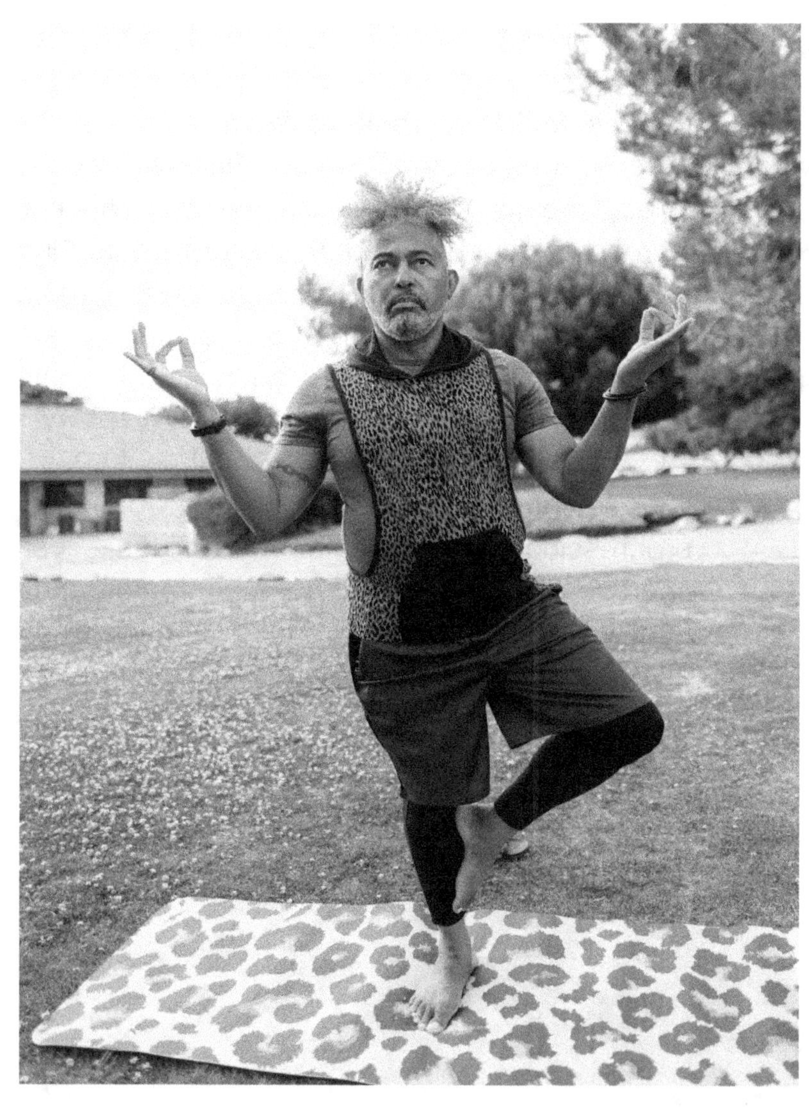

Chapter Four

Easy 6-minute Exercises

Step-by-step instructions for a variety of exercises targeting different muscle groups.

1. Push-Ups: Targets chest, shoulders, and triceps.
   - Place your hands shoulder-width apart and begin in the plank pose.
   - Lower body until chest nearly touches the ground.
   - Push up to return to your starting position.

2. Squats: Targets quadriceps, hamstrings, and glutes.
   - Stand with feet shoulder-width apart.
   - Lower hips back and down as if sitting in a chair.
   - Maintain a raised chest and knees behind the toes. Step back onto your heels to go back to standing.

3. Pull-Ups: Targets back, biceps, and shoulders.

   - Grip pull-up bar with hands slightly wider than shoulder-width.

   - Hang with arms fully extended.

   - Lift your torso till your chin touches the bar.

   - Lower back down with control.

4. Deadlifts: Targets hamstrings, glutes, lower back, and traps.

   - Stand with feet hip-width apart, barbell in front.

   - Hinge at hips, keeping back flat and chest up.

   - Grip barbell with hands just outside legs.

   - Drive through heels to stand up, keeping bar close to body.

5. Planks: Targets core muscles.

   - Start in a push-up position, but with elbows bent and forearms on the ground.

   -Maintain an erect posture from head to heels.

   - Hold for desired time, engaging core muscles.

6. Lunges: Targets quadriceps, hamstrings, glutes, and calves.

   - Stand with feet hip-width apart.

- Step forward with one leg and lower hips until both knees are bent at 90-degree angles.

- Keep the front knee behind the toes and the back knee hovering above the ground.

- Return to standing by pushing, then switch to the other leg.

Modifying exercises to accommodate various fitness levels and physical conditions

When modifying exercises to accommodate various fitness levels and physical conditions within the context of an Easy 6-minute Exercise for Fitness at 60+, consider:

1. **Low-Impact Options:** Offer alternatives to high-impact exercises, such as replacing jumping jacks with side steps or toe taps to reduce stress on joints.

2. **Adjusting Intensity:** Provide options to decrease or increase intensity, such as performing fewer or more repetitions, or using lighter or heavier weights based on individual abilities.

3. **Chair Modifications:** Incorporate seated exercises or exercises using a chair for support, such as seated leg lifts or seated arm curls, for those with mobility issues or balance concerns.

4. **Range of Motion:** Encourage participants to work within their comfortable range of motion,

emphasizing proper form over depth of movement to prevent injury and accommodate flexibility limitations.

5. Breathing and Rest: Emphasize the importance of proper breathing techniques and rest periods between exercises to maintain energy levels and prevent overexertion.

6. Personalization: Encourage participants to listen to their bodies and make modifications as needed, promoting a sense of autonomy and empowerment in their fitness journey.

By incorporating these modifications, individuals of varying fitness levels and physical conditions can safely and effectively participate in the Easy 6-minute Exercise for Fitness at 60+.

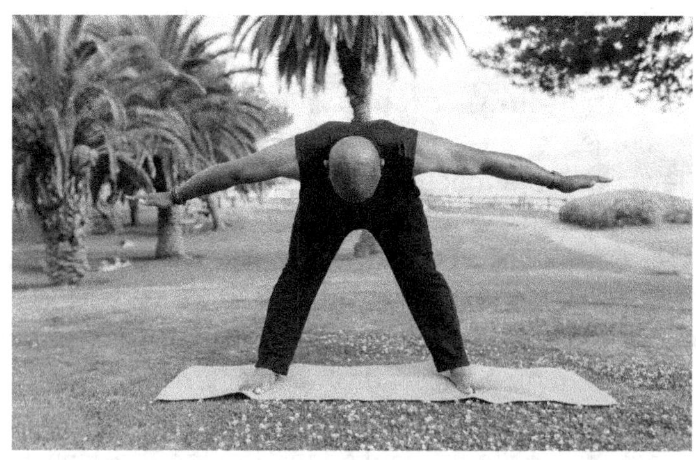

Chapter Five

Strategies for maintaining consistency in a fitness routine.

To maintain consistency in a fitness routine aligned with Easy 6-minute Exercise for Fitness at 60+, focus on setting achievable goals, scheduling workouts into your routine, varying exercises to prevent boredom, listening to your body for rest and recovery, seeking social support, and celebrating small victories to stay motivated.

Exploring the social aspects of staying active, such as group exercises or virtual classes.

Staying physically active holds numerous benefits for individuals over the age of 60, and integrating social elements into exercise routines can enhance both physical and mental well-being. Group exercises and virtual classes offer valuable avenues for social engagement while promoting fitness in this demographic.

1. Community Connection: Group exercises foster a sense of community among participants, providing opportunities for social interaction and support. Shared experiences during workouts create bonds that extend beyond the exercise session, potentially combating feelings of loneliness or isolation common among older adults.

2. Motivation and Accountability: Engaging in fitness activities with others encourages accountability and motivation. Group settings offer encouragement from peers and instructors, increasing adherence to exercise regimens. Virtual classes provide similar support networks through online communities, enabling individuals to connect regardless of geographical location.

3. Variety and Enjoyment: Group exercises and virtual classes offer a diverse range of activities tailored to different interests and fitness levels. From yoga and tai chi to dance and aerobics, participants can explore various options and find activities they enjoy, enhancing long-term adherence to exercise routines.

4. Cognitive Stimulation: Social interaction during physical activity stimulates cognitive function, contributing to overall brain health. Engaging in conversations, following instructions, and coordinating movements in a group setting or virtual class can sharpen cognitive skills and improve mental acuity.

5. Emotional Well-being: Regular social interaction through exercise positively impacts emotional well-being by reducing stress, anxiety, and depression. The camaraderie built in group exercises and virtual classes provides emotional support and a sense of belonging, fostering resilience against mental health challenges.

6. Adaptability and Accessibility: Virtual classes offer flexibility and accessibility, allowing individuals to participate from the comfort of their homes. This adaptability is particularly beneficial for older adults with mobility issues or those living in areas with limited access to fitness facilities.

Celebrating small victories and progress in overall health and fitness.

Celebrating small victories and progress in overall health and fitness is crucial, especially for individuals embarking on an Easy 6-minute Exercise for Fitness at 60+. Each step forward, no matter how small, is a testament to dedication and resilience. Whether it's mastering a new exercise, increasing endurance, or simply feeling more energized, these achievements deserve recognition. Embracing these milestones fosters motivation and keeps momentum going, ultimately leading to greater long-term success in maintaining health and fitness goals. So, rejoice in every small win, for they pave the way to a healthier, more vibrant life, even with just six minutes of exercise a day.

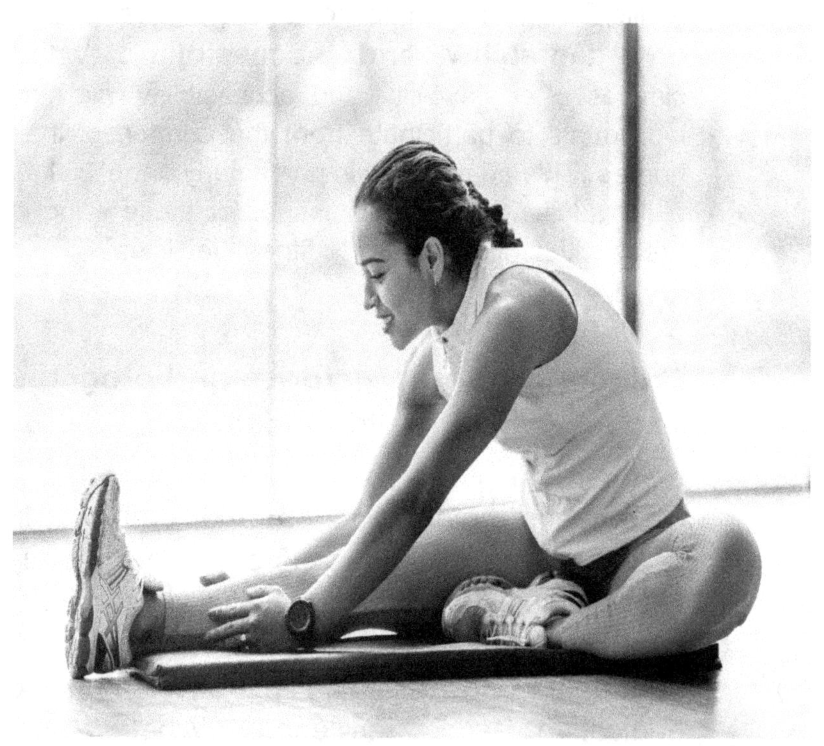

Chapter six

Nutrition and Hydration Tips

Guidance on maintaining a balanced diet to complement the exercise routine.

To maintain a balanced diet alongside the Easy 6-Minute Exercise for Fitness at 60+, ensure your meals are diverse and include a variety of food groups. Aim for a colorful plate with plenty of fruits and vegetables, which provide essential vitamins, minerals, and antioxidants. Incorporate lean proteins like poultry, fish, beans, and tofu to support muscle repair and growth. Opt for whole grains such as brown rice, quinoa, and oats to sustain energy levels throughout the day.

Additionally, prioritize healthy fats from sources like avocados, nuts, and olive oil, which can help reduce inflammation and support heart health. Stay hydrated by drinking plenty of water throughout the day, especially before and after exercising. Limit intake of processed foods, sugary snacks, and beverages high in added sugars and artificial ingredients.

Listen to your body's hunger and fullness cues, and eat mindfully to avoid overeating. Consider consulting with a registered dietitian or nutritionist to personalize your diet plan based on your specific needs and goals. Remember, consistency is key, so aim for gradual changes and sustainable habits for long-term health and fitness success.

The importance of hydration for older adults engaged in physical activity.

Certainly, here are some additional points highlighting the importance of hydration for older adults engaged in physical activity like the Easy 6-Minutes Exercise for Fitness at 60+:

1. **Optimal Muscle Function:** Hydration is essential for maintaining muscle function, which is particularly important for older adults to support mobility and independence. Proper hydration ensures that muscles receive an adequate supply of nutrients and oxygen, enhancing their ability to perform during exercise and reducing the risk of fatigue and injury.

2. Cognitive Function: Dehydration can impair cognitive function, leading to confusion, difficulty concentrating, and decreased coordination, which can compromise the safety and effectiveness of physical activity. By staying properly hydrated, older adults can maintain mental clarity and focus, allowing them to perform exercises with better form and technique.

3. Joint Health: Adequate hydration helps keep joints lubricated and flexible, reducing the risk of stiffness, discomfort, and injury during exercise. For older adults with arthritis or other joint issues, staying hydrated can alleviate symptoms and improve overall joint function, enabling them to engage in physical activity more comfortably and effectively.

4. Heart Health: Hydration plays a vital role in maintaining cardiovascular health, as proper fluid balance supports heart function and circulation. Older adults engaging in physical activity need sufficient hydration to support the increased demand on the heart and blood vessels, reducing the risk of cardiovascular complications such as elevated heart rate or blood pressure.

5. Temperature Regulation: During exercise, the body generates heat, and adequate hydration is necessary to regulate body temperature through sweat production and evaporation. Older adults may have a diminished ability to regulate body temperature, making them more susceptible to heat-related illnesses such as heat exhaustion or heat stroke. Staying hydrated helps older adults cool down more effectively during and after exercise, reducing the risk of overheating.

6. Digestive Health: Hydration is essential for maintaining proper digestion and nutrient absorption, which is crucial for older adults to support overall health and vitality. Drinking enough water helps prevent constipation and digestive discomfort, allowing older adults to feel more comfortable and energized during physical activity.

By prioritizing hydration alongside the Easy 6-Minutes Exercise for Fitness at 60+, older adults can enjoy improved performance, reduced risk of injury, and enhanced overall well-being, allowing them to keep up a busy and rewarding lifestyle as they get older.

Simple and practical nutritional advice for a healthy lifestyle.

Nutritional Advice for a Healthy Lifestyle at 60+:

1. A balanced diet should include eating a range of foods high in nutrients, such as fruits,

vegetables, whole grains, lean meats, and healthy fats.

2. Portion Control: To keep a healthy weight and avoid overindulging, pay attention to portion proportions.

3. Hydration: Stay adequately hydrated by drinking water throughout the day. Limit sugary drinks and alcohol intake.

4. Limit Processed Foods: Minimize intake of processed and packaged foods high in sodium, sugar, and unhealthy fats.

5. Fiber-Rich Foods: Incorporate fiber-rich foods like legumes, whole grains, fruits, and vegetables to support digestive health and regulate blood sugar levels.

6. Healthy Fats: Choose sources of healthy fats such as avocados, nuts, seeds, and olive oil to promote heart health and cognitive function.

7. Regular Meals: Aim for regular mealtimes to maintain stable energy levels and prevent excessive snacking.

8. Mindful Eating: Practice mindful eating by paying attention to hunger and fullness cues, savoring each bite, and avoiding distractions while eating.

Easy 6-Minute Exercise for Fitness at 60+:

1.Warm-Up (1 minute): Begin with gentle movements like arm circles, leg swings, and neck rotations to prepare the body for exercise.

2.Cardiovascular Exercise (2 minutes): Perform low-impact activities such as brisk walking, marching in place, or cycling on a stationary bike to elevate heart rate and improve circulation.

3.Strength Training (2 minutes): Incorporate bodyweight exercises like squats, lunges, push-ups, and chair dips to build muscle strength and improve balance.

4.Cool Down and Stretching (1 minute): Finish with gentle stretches targeting major muscle groups to enhance flexibility and prevent stiffness.

Consistency is key to reaping the benefits of both nutrition and exercise for a healthy lifestyle at 60+. Consult with a healthcare professional before starting any new exercise or dietary regimen, especially if you have pre-existing health conditions.

Chapter Seven

Overcoming Challenges

Addressing common obstacles to exercise, such as arthritis or mobility issues.

Addressing common obstacles to exercise, particularly for individuals aged 60 and above, necessitates a thoughtful approach that acknowledges and accommodates various physical limitations. Arthritis, for instance, can significantly impact joint mobility and cause discomfort during physical activity. In such cases, opting for exercises that are gentle on the joints, such as water aerobics or tai chi, can help maintain cardiovascular health and improve flexibility without exacerbating joint pain.

Mobility issues, whether due to age-related decline or specific health conditions, require tailored exercise routines that prioritize safety and effectiveness. Incorporating chair exercises, balance exercises, and resistance training using light weights or resistance bands can enhance muscle strength and stability while reducing the risk of falls.

Furthermore, emphasizing the importance of proper warm-up and cool-down routines becomes crucial in mitigating the risk of injury and promoting overall well-being. Stretching exercises targeted at improving flexibility and range of motion can help alleviate stiffness and enhance mobility, making daily activities more manageable and enjoyable.

Addressing nutrition and hydration needs is paramount for supporting overall health and fitness goals. Encouraging a balanced diet rich in nutrients essential for bone health, muscle function, and energy production can complement the benefits of regular exercise and support healthy aging.

Lastly, fostering a supportive and inclusive environment that encourages participation and celebrates progress can significantly motivate individuals to overcome obstacles and stay committed to their fitness journey. Group fitness classes tailored to older adults or seeking the guidance of certified fitness professionals experienced in working with seniors can provide invaluable support and encouragement along the way.

Tips for adapting exercises to accommodate individual limitations

Adapting exercises for individuals over 60 with limitations requires a personalized approach. Here are some tips:

1. Consultation: Prioritize a consultation with a healthcare professional to understand specific limitations and recommendations for safe exercise.

2. Modify Intensity: Reduce intensity levels based on individual capabilities, such as lowering weights or performing fewer repetitions.

3.Focus on Balance and Stability: Incorporate exercises that improve balance and stability, like standing on one leg or chair yoga poses.

4. Use Supportive Equipment: Utilize supportive equipment like chairs or resistance bands to aid in stability and reduce strain on joints.

5. Alternate Exercises: Offer alternative exercises targeting the same muscle groups to accommodate limitations while maintaining overall workout effectiveness.

6. Monitor Comfort Levels: Encourage individuals to listen to their bodies and adjust exercises accordingly to avoid discomfort or exacerbating existing limitations.

By implementing these strategies, individuals over 60 can safely engage in the Easy 6-Minute Exercise for Fitness while accommodating their individual limitations.

Encouragement for persisting through setbacks and challenges

Persisting through setbacks and challenges, especially when it comes to fitness, is crucial for maintaining a healthy and active lifestyle, especially for those aged 60 and above. Here's some encouragement tailored to that:

• Embrace Every Step of the Journey Every obstacle you face is a step closer to your ultimate objective. . Every challenge you overcome makes you stronger, both physically and mentally. Remember, progress is not always linear, but every effort you put in counts towards your overall well-being.

• Celebrate Your Victories

Even the smallest achievements deserve recognition. Whether it's completing a set of exercises or increasing the duration of your workout, celebrate your progress along the way. Recognize your progress and make use of it as inspiration to keep moving forward.

• Listen to Your Body

Your body knows best. Pay attention to how you feel during and after exercising. If something doesn't feel right, don't hesitate to adjust your routine or seek guidance from a professional. Rest when needed, but also challenge yourself when you're able to.

• Find Joy in Movement

Exercise doesn't have to be a chore. Explore different activities until you find what brings you joy. Whether it's dancing, swimming, or simply taking a brisk walk in nature, find ways to make fitness a fulfilling part of your life.

• Surround Yourself with support Surround yourself with individuals who believe in you and your ambitions. . Share your journey with friends, family, or a supportive community who can offer encouragement and accountability.You can conquer challenges and share your accomplishments together.

• Believe in Yourself

Above all, believe in your ability to overcome challenges and reach your fitness goals. Trust in your strength, resilience, and determination. With perseverance and a positive mindset, you can conquer any setback that comes your way.

Remember, you're never too old to prioritize your health and well-being. Every effort you invest in yourself is an investment in a happier, healthier future.

Keep pushing forward, and never underestimate the power of consistency and determination. You've got this!

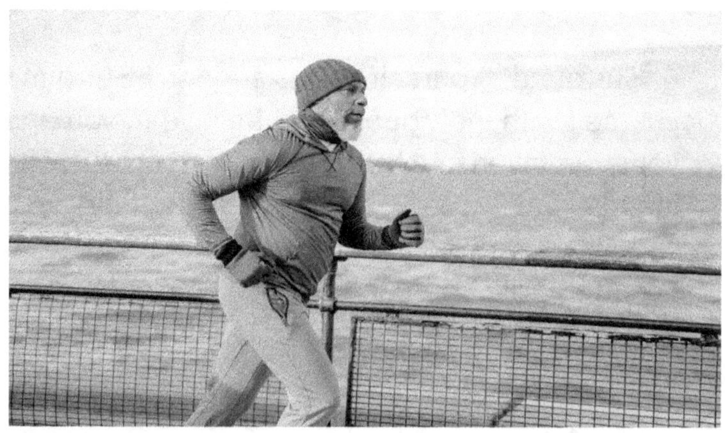

Conclusion

In conclusion, adopting a simple yet effective 6-minute exercise routine can significantly enhance fitness levels for individuals aged 60 and above. This accessible approach not only promotes physical well-being but also boosts mental clarity and overall quality of life. By prioritizing consistency and gradually increasing intensity, seniors can enjoy the countless benefits of staying active well into their golden years. Embracing this manageable exercise regimen empowers individuals to take charge of their health and age with vitality, proving that fitness knows no age limits.